The South Beach Diet

Ultimate Guide for Beginners with Healthy Recipes and Kick-Start Meal Plans

Emma Green

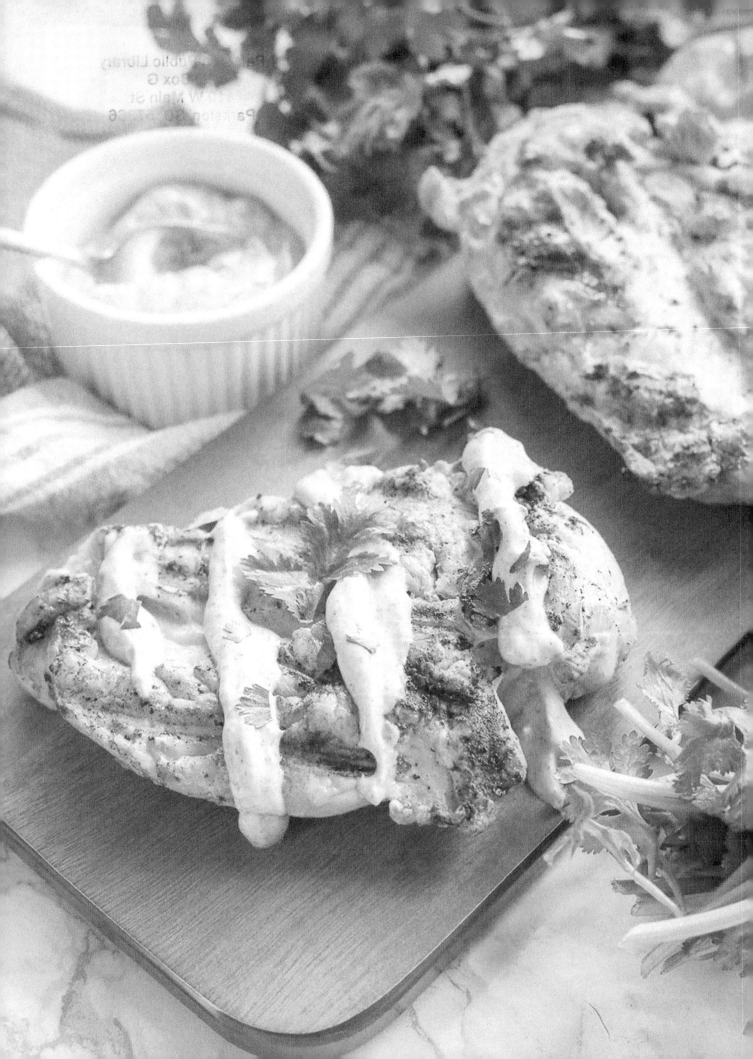

Disclaimer

The recipes and information in this book are provided for educational purposes only. Please always consult a licensed professional before making changes to your lifestyle or diet. The author and/or publisher shall have neither liability nor responsibility to anyone with respect to any loss or damage caused or alleged to be caused directly or indirectly by the information contained in this book. All trademarks and brands within this book are for clarifying purposes only and are owned by the owners themselves, not affiliated with this document.

Images from shutterstock.com

CONTENTS

Introduction

All the food we consume contains a large and wide number of nutrients. These can be divided into six general categories: water, proteins, carbohydrates (carbs), fats, vitamins, and minerals. The carbs and the fats can be both good and bad. Success in losing weight is found by preferring the best of each. That means lots of vegetables, fish, eggs, dairy, lean protein like chicken and turkey, whole grains, and nuts. The South Beach Diet is not high in carbohydrates but high in protein and healthy fats. The diet doesn't banish all carbs. The ones you do consume are low on the glycemic index (GI), an estimate of how carbs affect blood glucose.

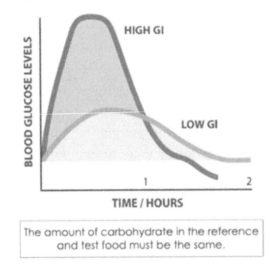

The amount of carbohydrate in the reference and test food must be the same.

Low-GI "good" carbs are known to keep your blood sugar and metabolism at healthy levels, and to keep you feeling fuller longer, while high-GI "bad" carbs have the opposite effect.

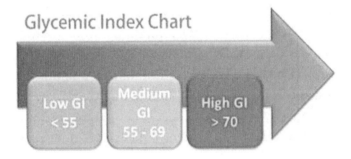

This book concentrates mostly on Phase I recipes as this phase is the most carb restrictive one. Practically any Phase I recipe can also be a Phase II recipe simply by serving it with additional carbs. For example you can eat guacamole with celery stalks on Phase I or add buttered toast for Phase II. You can add 1-2 diced carrots to any of your soups and it becomes Phase II friendly.

Phase I

The first phase of the South Beach Diet is two weeks long and rich in lean protein, low-fat dairy and high-fiber vegetables. During this phase you will be enjoying three normal well-balanced meals a day with snacks in between. At the same time this is the most carb restrictive phase and it eliminates cravings. The foods you will not be enjoying throughout the first phase are the following:

- **Fruit**: All kinds of fruits including dried fruit and fruit juices are to be avoided in this stage.
- **Vegetables**: Carrots, beets, potatoes, green peas, corn, turnip, or other starchy vegetables are to cut out.
- **Starches:** Bread, pastries, pasta, rice, cereal, oatmeal, matzo are out of the question.
- **Meat and poultry:** Fatty cuts like brisket or rib steaks, dark meat poultry products, duck, and ham are also to be avoided.
- **Dairy:** no whole or 2% milk.
- **All alcohol beverages** are restricted.
- **Sweets**: Candies and treats containing sugar as well as ice cream are eliminated.

Allowed vegetables chart

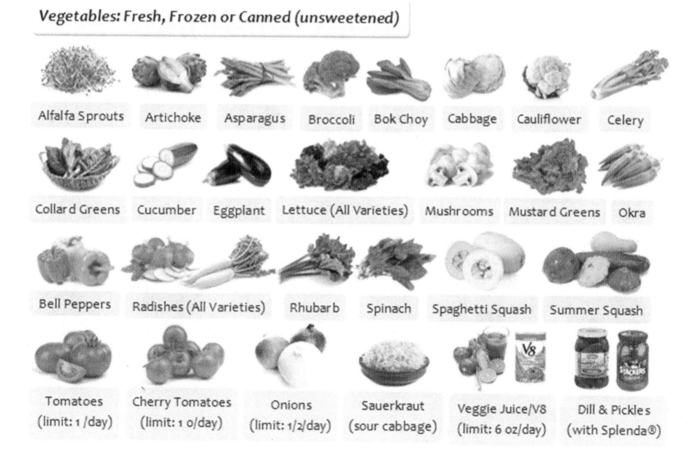

Vegetables: Fresh, Frozen or Canned (unsweetened)

Alfalfa Sprouts | Artichoke | Asparagus | Broccoli | Bok Choy | Cabbage | Cauliflower | Celery

Collard Greens | Cucumber | Eggplant | Lettuce (All Varieties) | Mushrooms | Mustard Greens | Okra

Bell Peppers | Radishes (All Varieties) | Rhubarb | Spinach | Spaghetti Squash | Summer Squash

Tomatoes (limit: 1 /day) | Cherry Tomatoes (limit: 1 o/day) | Onions (limit: 1/2/day) | Sauerkraut (sour cabbage) | Veggie Juice/V8 (limit: 6 oz/day) | Dill & Pickles (with Splenda®)

Allowed legumes

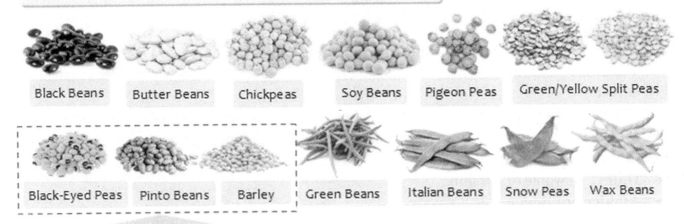

Beans & Legumes: Fresh, Frozen or Canned (unsweetened)

Black Beans | Butter Beans | Chickpeas | Soy Beans | Pigeon Peas | Green/Yellow Split Peas

Black-Eyed Peas | Pinto Beans | Barley | Green Beans | Italian Beans | Snow Peas | Wax Beans

ONLY ALLOWED IN **PHASE 2**

Allowed sauces and seasonings

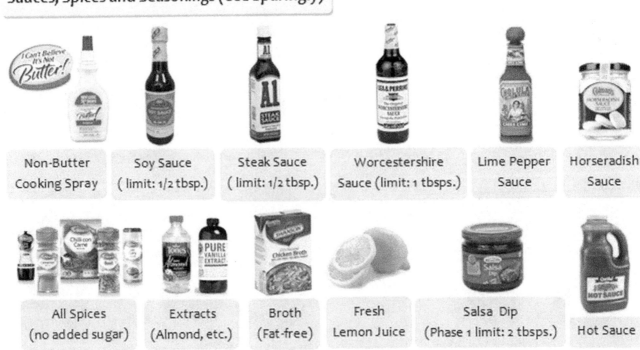

Sauces, Spices and Seasonings (Use Sparingly)

Non-Butter Cooking Spray | Soy Sauce (limit: 1/2 tbsp.) | Steak Sauce (limit: 1/2 tbsp.) | Worcestershire Sauce (limit: 1 tbsps.) | Lime Pepper Sauce | Horseradish Sauce

All Spices (no added sugar) | Extracts (Almond, etc.) | Broth (Fat-free) | Fresh Lemon Juice | Salsa Dip (Phase 1 limit: 2 tbsps.) | Hot Sauce

Allowed meat chart

Beef: Lean cuts

Top Round   Eye of Round   Tenderloin   Top Loin

Ground Beef
(extra lean 96/4, lean 92/8, sirloin 90/10)

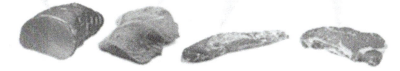
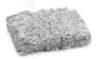

Lamb: All visible fat removed

Loin   Center Cut   Loin Chop

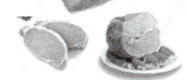
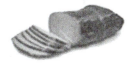

Lunchmeat: Fat-free or Low-fat

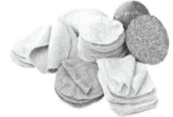

Pork

Tenderloin   Canadian Bacon

Loin   Boiled Ham

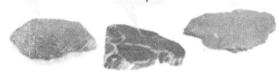

Veal

Top Round   Chop   Leg Cutlets

Meat Products: <3gms fat per 3-oz portion

Bacon   Burger   Sausage Patties

Hotdog

Seafood: All fish & Shellfish

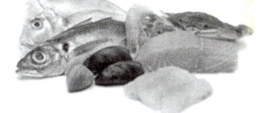

Bacon: Limit to 2 slices per day

Sausage Pattie : Limit to 1 patty per day

Phase I Meal Plan

Day 1	
Breakfast	Chicken Salad in Cucumber Cups *(recipe on p. 25)* Fresh tomato juice with salt and pepper
Snack	Celery and cucumber sticks with hummus *(recipe on p. 31)*
Lunch	Grilled chicken breast with Indian spices
Snack	Roasted nuts (15 almonds/30 pistachios)
Dinner	Home-style dal *(recipe on p.38)* 1 stick mozzarella

Day 2	
Breakfast	Hard-boiled eggs with boiled ham Decaffeinated tea or coffee
Snack	Turkey roll-ups *(recipe on p. 57)*
Lunch	Indian style cauliflower soup *(recipe on p. 35)*
Snack	Roasted nuts (15 almonds/30 pistachios)
Dinner	2 fillets pecan-crusted cod with spinach *(recipe on p. 45)*

Day 3	
Breakfast	1 slice quiche with spinach, mushrooms and bell peppers Fresh tomato juice with salt and pepper
Snack	Guacamole *(recipe on p.32)*
Lunch	Pesto chicken breast *(recipe on p. 58)*
Snack	Roasted nuts (15 almonds/30 pistachios)
Dinner	Bok choy shrimp with stir-fried yellow squash *(recipe on p.49)*

Day 4	
Breakfast	Omelet with chopped mushrooms 8 oz fat free milk

Snack	Roasted nuts (15 almonds/30 pistachios)
Lunch	Chicken kale soup *(recipe on p. 36)*
Snack	Cherry tomato salad *(recipe on p. 18)*
Dinner	Ground turkey salad *(recipe on p. 19)*
Day 5	
Breakfast	1 slice Quiche Lorraine *(recipe on p. 27)* Fresh tomato juice with salt and pepper
Snack	Roasted nuts (15 almonds/30 pistachios)
Lunch	Spinach soup *(recipe on p. 37)* Cabbage stir-fry with Indian spices
Snack	Celery sticks with Cilantro Dip *(recipe on p. 34)*
Dinner	Baked chicken Cordon Bleu *(recipe on p. 59)*

Phase II

The aim of the second phase of the South Beach Diet is to define your personally correct carb level and reach your personal target weight. The phase is strictly individual and may be of different lengths for different people. It may be broken into six weeks during which you gradually restore your carbs:

Week 1. The plan of the first week of Phase II is to eat one serving of a carbohydrate food each day, experimenting to see how you feel. This will be a serving of fresh fruit for either breakfast or lunch or dinner.

Week 2. This week you will be enjoying each day one serving of fresh fruit plus one serving of high-fiber starchy foods, e.g. beans or other legumes.

Week 3. This week again another serving per day of carbs will be added and bread can be an option. It is better to choose bread with more fiber and less starch.

Week 4. Add another serving of carbohydrate food.

Week 5. Add one more serving of carbs.

Week 6. Add another serving of cards and by this time you will be having three servings of fruit and three servings of grains or starches each day.

Going through the second phase implies slow weight loss and will last as long as it takes you to lose your desired weight.

Phase II Meal Plan

Day 1

Breakfast	1 slice cheddar broccoli quiche (recipe on p. 28)
Snack	1 container strawberries
Lunch	Tuna salad (recipe on p. 14)
Snack	Turkey deli meat with cucumber slices
Dinner	Ground turkey lettuce wraps (recipe on p. 64)

Day 2

Breakfast	1 slice Parmesan kale quiche *(recipe on p. 30)*
Snack	Greek yogurt with blueberries
Lunch	Split pea soup with Italian sausage *(recipe on p. 40)*
Snack	Celery sticks with cilantro dip *(recipe on p. 34)*
Dinner	Balsamic salmon *(recipe on p.46)*

Day 3

Breakfast	Fresh pineapple with cottage cheese
Snack	Greek yogurt
Lunch	Chinese hot and sour soup *(recipe on p. 43)*
Snack	Celery sticks with white bean dip *(recipe on p. 33)*
Dinner	Asian marinade kebabs *(recipe on p. 65)*

Day 4

Breakfast	1 slice feta spinach quiche *(recipe on p. 29)*
Snack	1 banana
Lunch	Egg soup *(recipe on p. 42)*
Snack	Salmon cucumber bites *(recipe on p. 55)*
Dinner	Spinach stuffed chicken *(recipe on p. 68)*

Day 5	
Breakfast	Fresh strawberries with cottage cheese
Snack	1 cup soy milk
Lunch	Gazpacho *(recipe on p. 39)*
Snack	Cherry tomato salad *(recipe on p. 18)*
Dinner	Greek style chicken *(recipe on p. 61)*

Phase III

Phase III of the South Beach diet is meant for weight maintenance. No food is off limits here as long as you maintain your correct weight. You are still encouraged to eat "good" carbs, such as whole-grain bread, brown rice, whole-wheat pasta and fruit, but they are already in your lifestyle once you get to this phase. Your diet has definitely become greener, however you can enjoy indulging in a special, decadent treat on occasion. Live every day to the fullest— in moderation.

Pros & Cons

Pros:

- Enhances heart health
- Boosts weight loss
- Reduces hunger
- Stabilizes blood sugar level

Cons:

- Forbids some healthy, beneficial fats
- Encourages Omega 6 vegetable oils
- Permits artificial sweeteners

Salads

Tuna salad (Phase I)

Prep time: 10 minutes

Cooking time: none

Servings: 3

Nutrition facts per serving:

Calories 212

Total carbs 4.8 g

Protein 14.3 g

Total sugars 1.1 g

Ingredients:

- 1 can tuna (6 oz)
- 1/3 cup fresh cucumber, chopped
- 1/3 cup fresh tomato, chopped
- 1/3 cup avocado, chopped
- 1/3 cup celery, chopped
- 2 garlic cloves, minced
- 4 tsp olive oil
- 2 tbsp lime juice
- Pinch of black pepper

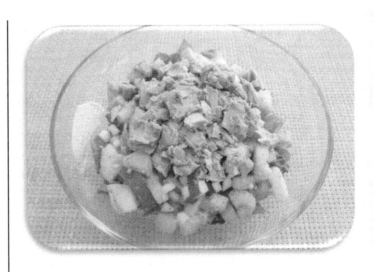

Instructions:

1. Prepare the dressing by combining olive oil, lime juice, minced garlic and black pepper.
2. Mix the salad ingredients in a salad bowl and drizzle with the dressing.

Roasted Portobello Salad (Phase I)

Prep time: 10 minutes

Cooking time: none

Servings: 4

Nutrition facts per serving:

Calories 501

Total carbs 22.3 g

Protein 14.9 g

Total sugars 2.1 g

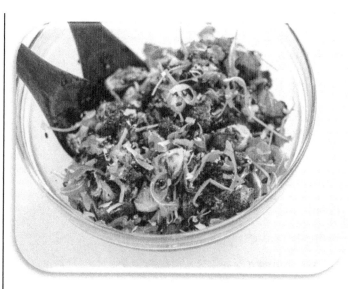

Ingredients:

- 1½ lb Portobello mushrooms, stems trimmed
- 3 heads Belgian endive, sliced
- 1 small red onion, sliced
- 4 oz blue cheese
- 8 oz mixed salad greens

Dressing:

- 3 tbsp red wine vinegar
- 1 tbsp Dijon mustard
- 2/3 cup olive oil
- Salt and pepper to taste

Instructions:

1. Preheat the oven to 450°F.
2. Prepare the dressing by whisking together vinegar, mustard, salt and pepper. Slowly add olive oil while whisking.
3. Cut the mushrooms and arrange them on a baking sheet, stem-side up. Coat the mushrooms with some dressing and bake for 15 minutes.
4. In a salad bowl toss the salad greens with onion, endive and cheese. Sprinkle with the dressing.
5. Add mushrooms to the salad bowl.

Shredded chicken salad (Phase I)

Prep time: 5 minutes

Cooking time: 10 minutes

Servings: 6

Nutrition facts per serving:

Calories 117

Total carbs 9 g

Protein 11.6 g

Total sugars 4.2 g

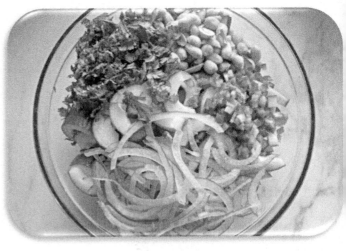

Ingredients:

- 2 chicken breasts, boneless, skinless
- 1 head iceberg lettuce, cut into strips
- 2 bell peppers, cut into strips
- 1 fresh cucumber, quartered, sliced
- 3 scallions, sliced
- 2 tbsp chopped peanuts
- 1 tbsp peanut vinaigrette
- Salt to taste
- 1 cup water

Instructions:

1. In a skillet simmer one cup of salted water.
2. Add the chicken breasts, cover and cook on low for 5 minutes. Remove the cover. Then remove the chicken from the skillet and shred with a fork.
3. In a salad bowl mix the vegetables with the cooled chicken, season with salt and sprinkl with peanut vinaigrette and chopped peanuts.

Broccoli Salad (Phase I)

Prep time: 10 minutes

Cooking time: none

Servings: 6

Nutrition facts per serving:

Calories 220

Total carbs 17.3 g

Protein 11 g

Total sugars 10 g

Ingredients:

- 1 medium head broccoli, raw, florets only
- ½ cup red onion, chopped
- 12 oz turkey bacon, chopped, fried until crisp
- ½ cup cherry tomatoes, halved
- ¼ cup sunflower kernels
- ¾ cup raisins
- ¾ cup mayonnaise
- 2 tbsp white vinegar

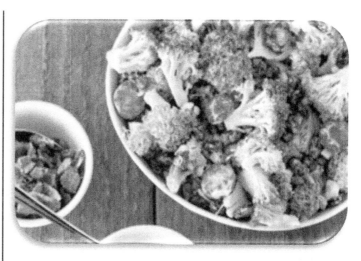

Instructions:

1. In a salad bowl combine the broccoli, tomatoes and onion.
2. Mix mayo with vinegar and sprinkle over the broccoli.
3. Add the sunflower kernels, raisins and bacon and toss well.

Cherry Tomato Salad (Phase I)

Prep time: 10 minutes

Cooking time: none

Servings: 6

Nutrition facts per serving:

Calories 259

Total carbs 10.7 g

Protein 2.4 g

Total sugars 3.6 g

Ingredients:

- 40 cherry tomatoes, halved
- 1 cup mozzarella balls, halved
- 1 cup green olives, sliced
- 1 can (6 oz) black olives, sliced
- 2 green onions, chopped
- 3 oz roasted pine nuts

Dressing:

- ½ cup olive oil
- 2 tbsp red wine vinegar
- 1 tsp dried oregano
- Salt and pepper to taste

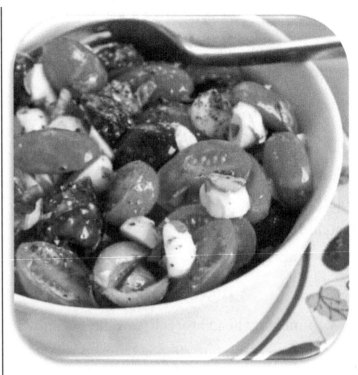

Instructions:

1. In a salad bowl, combine the tomatoes, olives and onions.
2. Prepare the dressing by combining olive oil with red wine vinegar, dried oregano, salt and pepper.
3. Sprinkle with the dressing and add the nuts.
4. Let marinate in the fridge for 1 hour.

Ground turkey salad (Phase I)

Prep time: 10 minutes

Cooking time: 35 minutes

Servings: 6

Nutrition facts per serving:

Calories 176

Total carbs 9.1 g

Protein 17.8 g

Total sugars 2.5 g

Ingredients:

- 1 lb lean ground turkey
- ½ inch ginger, minced
- 2 garlic cloves, minced
- 1 onion, chopped
- 1 tbsp olive oil
- 1 bag lettuce leaves (for serving)
- ¼ cup fresh cilantro, chopped
- 2 tsp coriander powder
- 1 tsp red chili powder
- 1 tsp turmeric powder
- Salt to taste
- 4 cups water

Dressing:

- 2 tbsp fat free yogurt
- 1 tbsp sour cream, non-fat
- 1 tbsp low fat mayonnaise
- 1 lemon, juiced
- 1 tsp red chili flakes
- Salt and pepper to taste

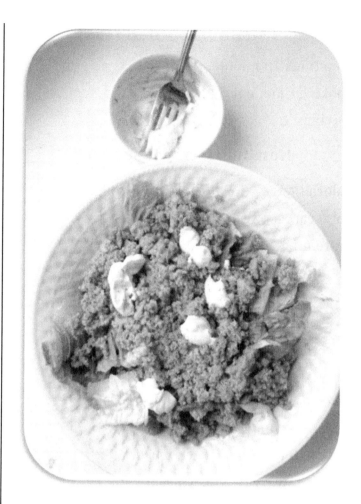

Instructions:

1. In a skillet sauté the garlic and ginger in olive oil for 1 minute. Add onion and season with salt. Cook for 10 minutes over medium heat.

2. Add the ground turkey and sauté for 3 more minutes. Add the spices (turmeric, red chili powder and coriander powder).

3. Add 4 cups water and cook for 30 minutes, covered.

4. Prepare the dressing by combining yogurt, sour cream, mayo, lemon juice, chili flakes, salt and pepper.

5. To serve arrange the salad leaves on serving plates and place the cooked ground turkey on them. Top with dressing.

Asian Cucumber Salad (Phase I)

Prep time: 10 minutes

Cooking time: none

Servings: 6

Nutrition facts per serving:

Calories 52

Total carbs 5.7 g

Protein 1 g

Total sugars 3.1 g

Ingredients:

- 1 lb cucumbers, sliced
- 2 scallions, sliced
- 2 tbsp sliced pickled ginger, chopped
- ¼ cup cilantro
- ½ red jalapeño, chopped
- 3 tbsp rice wine vinegar
- 1 tbsp sesame oil
- 1 tbsp sesame seeds

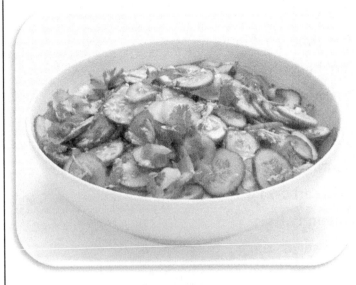

Instructions:

1. In a salad bowl combine all ingredients and toss together.

Cauliflower Tofu Salad (Phase I)

Prep time: 10 minutes

Cooking time: 15 minutes

Servings: 4

Nutrition facts per serving:

Calories 328

Total carbs 34.1 g

Protein 11.1 g

Total sugars 11.5 g

Ingredients:

- 2 cups cauliflower florets, blended
- 1 fresh cucumber, diced
- ½ cup green olives, diced
- 1/3 cup red onion, diced
- 2 tbsp toasted pine nuts
- 2 tbsp raisins
- 1/3 cup feta, crumbled
- ½ cup pomegranate seeds
- 2 lemons (juiced, zest grated)
- 8 oz tofu
- 2 tsp oregano
- 2 garlic cloves, minced
- ½ tsp red chili flakes
- 3 tbsp olive oil
- Salt and pepper to taste

Instructions:

1. Season the processed cauliflower with salt and transfer to a strainer to drain.

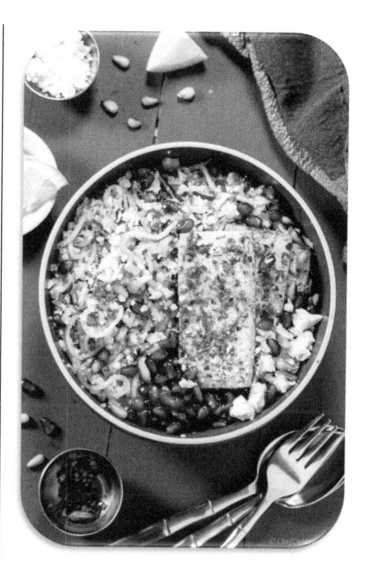

2. Prepare the marinade for tofu by combining 2 tbsp lemon juice, 1.5 tbsp olive oil, minced garlic, chili flakes, oregano, salt and pepper. Coat tofu in the marinade and set aside.
3. Preheat the oven to 450°F.
4. Bake tofu on a baking sheet for 12 minutes.
5. In a salad bowl mix the remaining marinade with onions, cucumber, cauliflower, olives and raisins. Add in the remaining olive oil and grated lemon zest.
6. Top with tofu, pine nuts, feta and pomegranate seeds.

Scallop Caesar Salad (Phase I/II)

Prep time: 5 minutes

Cooking time: 2 minutes

Servings: 2

Nutrition facts per serving:

Calories 340

Total carbs 14 g

Protein 30.7 g

Total sugars 2.2 g

Ingredients:

- 8 sea scallops
- 4 cups romaine lettuce
- 2 tsp olive oil
- 3 tbsp Caesar Salad Dressing
- 1 tsp lemon juice
- Salt and pepper to taste

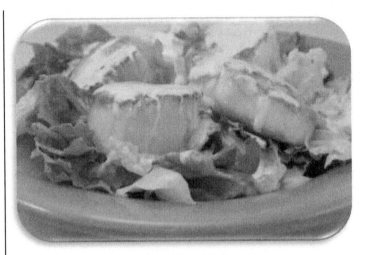

Instructions:

1. In a frying pan heat olive oil and cook the scallops in one layer no longer than 2 minutes per both sides. Season with salt and pepper to taste.
2. Arrange lettuce on plates and place scallops on top.
3. Pour over the Caesar dressing and lemon juice.

Chicken Avocado Salad (Phase I/II)

Prep time: 30 minutes

Cooking time: 15 minutes

Servings: 4

Nutrition facts per serving:

Calories 380

Total carbs 10 g

Protein 38 g

Total sugars 11.5 g

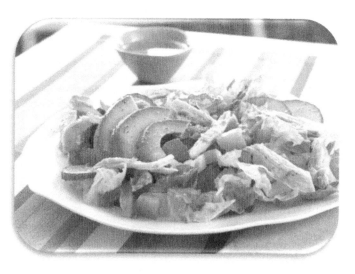

Ingredients:

- 1 lb chicken breast, cooked, shredded
- 1 avocado, pitted, peeled, sliced
- 2 tomatoes, diced
- 1 cucumber, peeled, sliced
- 1 head lettuce, chopped
- 3 tbsp olive oil
- 2 tbsp lime juice
- 1 tbsp cilantro, chopped
- Salt and pepper to taste

Instructions:

1. In a bowl whisk together oil, lime juice, cilantro, salt, and a pinch of pepper.
2. Combine lettuce, tomatoes, cucumber in a salad bowl and toss with half of the dressing.
3. Toss chicken with the remaining dressing and combine with vegetable mixture.
4. Top with avocado.

California Wraps (Phase I/II)

Prep time: 5 minutes

Cooking time: 15 minutes

Servings: 4

Nutrition facts per serving:

Calories 140

Total carbs 4 g

Protein 9 g

Total sugars 0.5 g

Ingredients:

- 4 slices turkey breast, cooked
- 4 slices ham, cooked
- 4 lettuce leaves
- 4 slices tomato
- 4 slices avocado
- 1 tsp lime juice
- A handful watercress leaves
- 4 tbsp Ranch dressing, sugar free

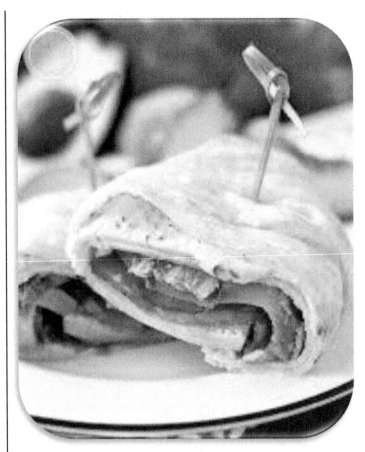

Instructions:

1. Top a lettuce leaf with turkey slice, ham slice and tomato.
2. In a bowl combine avocado and lime juice and place on top of tomatoes. Top with water cress and dressing.
3. Repeat with the remaining ingredients for 4. Topping each lettuce leaf with a turkey slice, ham slice, tomato and dressing.

Chicken Salad in Cucumber Cups (Phase I)

Prep time: 5 minutes

Cooking time:15 minutes

Servings: 4

Nutrition facts per serving:

Calories 116

Total carbs 4 g

Protein 12 g

Total sugars 0.5 g

Ingredients:

- ½ chicken breast, skinless, boiled and shredded
- 2 long cucumbers, cut into 8 thick rounds each, scooped out (won't use in a recipe).
- 1 tsp ginger, minced
- 1 tsp lime zest, grated
- 4 tsp olive oil
- 1 tsp sesame oil
- 1 tsp lime juice
- Salt and pepper to taste

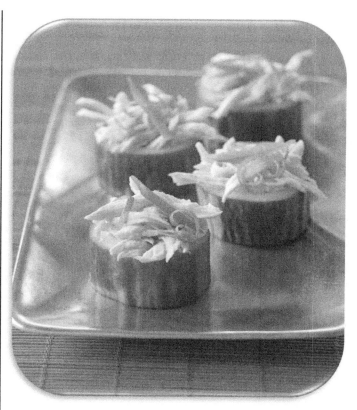

Instructions:

1. In a bowl combine lime zest, juice, olive and sesame oils, ginger, season with salt.
2. Toss the chicken with the dressing and fill the cucumber cups with the salad.

Quiches & Dips

Quiche with spinach, mushrooms and bell peppers (Phase I/II)

Prep time: 10 minutes

Cooking time: 1 hour

Servings: 6-8

Nutrition facts per serving:

Calories 138

Total carbs 7.5 g

Protein 16 g

Total sugars 3.4 g

Ingredients:

- 8 eggs
- ¼ cup milk, fat free
- 1 cup cottage cheese, low fat
- 2 cups any low fat cheese, grated
- 1 garlic, minced
- 2 cups spinach
- 3 cups mushrooms to your liking, diced
- 1 bell pepper, diced
- 1 cup red onions, diced
- 1 tsp red chili powder
- 1 tsp garam masala
- 1 tbsp olive oil
- Salt and pepper to taste

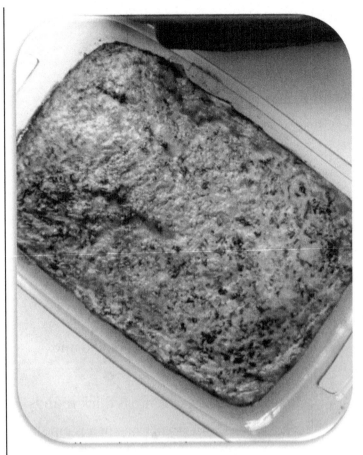

Instructions:

1. Beat the eggs with milk, add the cottage cheese and stir.
2. In a skillet sauté the garlic in the olive oil for about 30 seconds. Add the onions. Season with chili powder and garam masala.
3. Add the bell peppers, mushrooms and cook for 5 minutes. Add the spinach and sauté until wilted.
4. Preheat the oven to 375°F.
5. Spray a baking pan with some oil. Layer the sautéed vegetables, then the cheese. Pour the egg mixture over the pan making sure the liquid has evenly coated the vegetables.
6. Bake for 45 minutes.

Quiche Lorraine (Phase II)

Prep time: 10 minutes

Cooking time: 40 minutes

Servings: 6-8

Nutrition facts per serving:

Calories 372

Total carbs 5.7 g

Protein 25.6 g

Total sugars 2 g

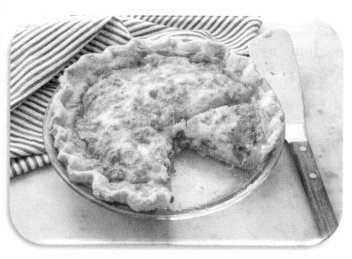

Ingredients:

- 8 eggs
- 1 cup half and half
- ¼ cup bell pepper, diced, roasted
- 12 oz Swiss cheese, shredded
- 12 oz turkey bacon, crumbled
- 1 tsp parsley flakes
- ¼ tsp ground nutmeg
- Salt and pepper to taste

Instructions:

1. Preheat the oven to 350°F.
2. In a bowl mix eggs, half peppers and spices. Add the cheese and crumbled bacon.
3. Grease a baking pan and pour in the mixture. Bake for 40 minutes.

Cheddar Broccoli Quiche (Phase I)

Prep time: 10 minutes

Cooking time: 50 minutes

Servings: 6

Nutrition facts per serving:

Calories 128

Total carbs 4.8 g

Protein 15 g

Total sugars 2 g

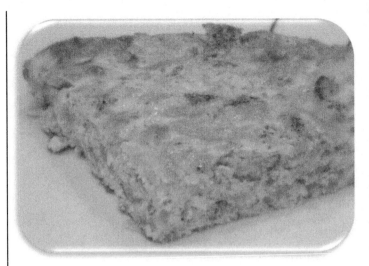

Ingredients:

- 2 cups egg beaters
- ½ cup cottage cheese, low fat
- ½ cup Cheddar, low fat, shredded
- ¼ cup onion, chopped
- 10 oz broccoli, chopped
- 1 tsp olive oil
- Salt and pepper to taste

Instructions:

1. Preheat the oven to 350°F.
2. In a skillet sauté onions in olive oil for 5 minutes, stirring. Add the broccoli and mix well.
3. Arrange broccoli and onions in a sprayed baking dish.
4. Mix the remaining ingredients until well blended and pour over the broccoli.
5. Bake for 50 minutes.

Feta Spinach Quiche (Phase I)

Prep time: 10 minutes

Cooking time: 25 minutes

Servings: 6

Nutrition facts per serving:

Calories 134

Total carbs 13.7 g

Protein 10.3 g

Total sugars 2 g

Ingredients:

- ½ cup egg beaters
- 2 eggs
- 1 1/3 cups milk, low fat
- ½ cup feta cheese
- 1 onion, diced
- 8 oz baby spinach
- Salt and pepper to taste

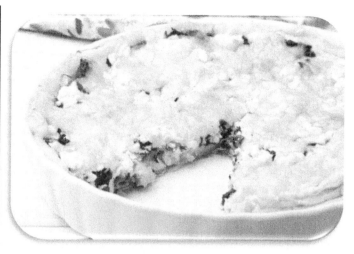

Instructions:

1. In a skillet sauté onions in olive oil, stirring, for 5 minutes. Add the spinach and cook until wilted.
2. In a bowl whisk together eggs, egg beaters and milk. Add the spinach and onion mixture. Season with salt and pepper.
3. Preheat oven to 400°F.
4. Pour the quiche mixture into a greased baking dish. Top with feta.
5. Bake for 25 minutes.

Parmesan Kale Quiche (Phase I)

Prep time: 10 minutes

Cooking time: 40 minutes

Servings: 6-8

Nutrition facts per serving:

Calories 119

Total carbs 5.4 g

Protein 9.8 g

Total sugars 2 g

Ingredients:

- 2 eggs
- 1 bunch kale, ripped into small pieces
- ¼ cup sun-dried tomatoes, chopped
- 1 onion, chopped
- 1 cup cottage cheese
- ¾ cup Parmesan, grated
- 1 tbsp olive oil
- 1 tsp Dijon mustard
- 1 tbsp Italian seasoning

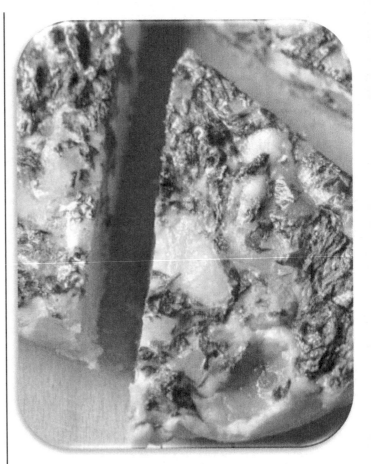

Instructions:

1. In a skillet sauté onions in olive oil, stirring, for 5 minutes. Add the kale and cook until wilted.
2. In a bowl whisk together eggs, cottage cheese, seasoning, mustard and Parmesan. Mix into the vegetables.
3. Preheat the oven to 375°F.
4. Pour the quiche mixture into a greased baking dish and bake for 40 minutes.

Plain Hummus (Phase I)

Prep time: overnight

Cooking time: 40 minutes

Servings: 4

Nutrition facts per serving:

Calories 340

Total carbs 21.7 g

Protein 10.1 g

Total sugars 5.9 g

Ingredients:

- 1/2 lb chickpeas, soaked overnight
- 5 garlic cloves, minced
- 3 tbsp tahini paste
- 2 tbsp olive oil
- 2 tbsp lemon juice
- 1-2 tsp paprika powder
- 2 tsp mint, chopped
- Salt to taste
- 3 cups water

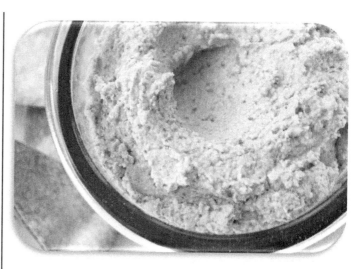

Instructions:

1. Prepare the soaked chickpeas by boiling in 3 cups of water until soft.
2. Grind the chickpeas together with garlic and olive oil.
3. Add the tahini paste and lemon juice. Season with salt and pepper.
4. Add the mint and mix well.
5. Store in the fridge and serve cold.

Avocado Guacamole (Phase I)

Prep time: 5 minutes

Cooking time: 3 minutes

Servings: 4

Nutrition facts per serving:

Calories 48

Total carbs 4.2 g

Protein 2 g

Total sugars 1.7 g

Ingredients:

- 1/3 avocado, peeled, mashed
- 1/3 cup cottage cheese, low fat
- 1 onion, chopped
- 1 garlic clove, minced
- ¼ cup cilantro, chopped
- 2 tbsp lemon juice
- ¼ tsp lemon zest, grated
- Salt and pepper to taste
- Celery sticks for serving

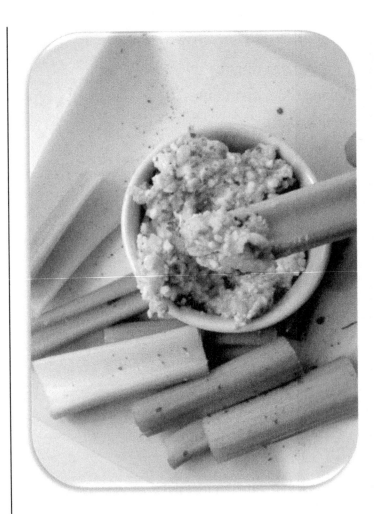

Instructions:

1. Mix all ingredients well and store in the fridge. Serve cool with celery sticks.

Note: can be enjoyed with whole wheat bread/crackers on Phase II

White bean dip (Phase I)

Prep time: 5 minutes

Cooking time:10 minutes

Servings: 4

Nutrition facts per serving:

Calories 179

Total carbs 22.2 g

Protein 7.5 g

Total sugars 0.4 g

Ingredients:

- 14 oz can white beans, rinsed
- 2 garlic cloves, chopped
- 10 black olives, pitted, chopped
- 2 tbsp parsley, chopped
- 2 tbsp olive oil
- 1½ tbsp lemon juice
- ¼ tsp dried oregano
- Pepper to taste

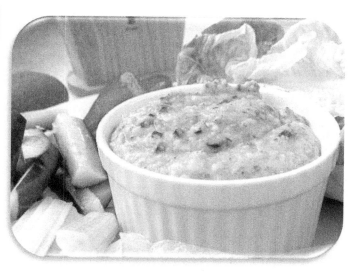

Instructions:

1. In a food processor purée the beans, garlic, parsley, oregano, lemon juice, olive oil and black pepper.
2. Transfer to a bowl, add olives and mix well.
3. Serve with celery or cucumber sticks.
   Note: can be enjoyed with pita bread for Phase II

Cilantro Dip (Phase I/II)

Prep time: 5 minutes

Cooking time:5 minutes

Servings: 8

Nutrition facts per serving:

Calories 100

Total carbs 1 g

Protein 1 g

Total sugars 0.4 g

Ingredients:

- 1 bunch cilantro, stems intact
- 1 garlic clove
- 1/3 cup walnuts, toasted
- 3 tbsp sour cream, reduced fat
- ¼ cup olive oil
- 2 tsp lemon juice
- Salt and pepper to taste

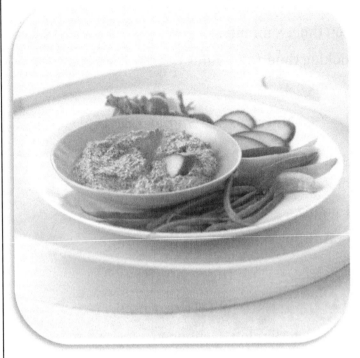

Instructions:

1. In a food processor purée the cilantro, garlic and walnuts.
2. Add oil, sour cream, lemon juice and season with salt and pepper. Pulse to combine.

Soups

Cauliflower Soup Indian Style (Phase I)

Prep time: 10 minutes

Cooking time: 40 minutes

Servings: 4

Nutrition facts per serving:

Calories 155

Total carbs 18.5 g

Protein 7.5 g

Total sugars 5.8 g

Ingredients:

- 1 head cauliflower, cut into florets
- 1 onion, chopped
- 1 garlic clove, minced
- ½ inch ginger, minced
- ½ cup fresh cilantro, chopped
- 1 cup sour cream, fat free
- 2 tsp coriander powder
- 1 tsp chili powder
- Pinch of garam masala
- 1 tbsp olive oil
- 3 cups chicken stock or water

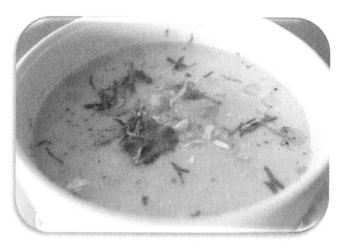

Instructions:

1. In a skillet sauté garlic and ginger in olive oil for about 40 seconds. add the onion and cook for 5 minutes. Season with coriander and chili powders.
2. Add the cauliflower and mix well.
3. Pour in the chicken stock or water and bring to a boil.
4. Cook for 20 minutes.
5. Transfer to a food processor and blend until smooth. Add sour cream and garam masala and pulse.
6. Serve with fresh cilantro.

Note: can be enjoyed with whole wheat crackers on Phase II.

Chicken Kale Soup (Phase I)

Prep time: 10 minutes

Cooking time: 40 minutes

Servings: 4

Nutrition facts per serving:

Calories 155

Total carbs 18.5 g

Protein 7.5 g

Total sugars 5.8 g

Ingredients:

- 3 cups chicken broth
- 1 cup chicken breast, skinless and boneless, cubed
- 1 bunch kale, chopped
- 1 cup red onion, diced
- 2 garlic cloves, minced
- 2 tsp red chili flakes
- 1 tsp thyme
- Salt and pepper to taste

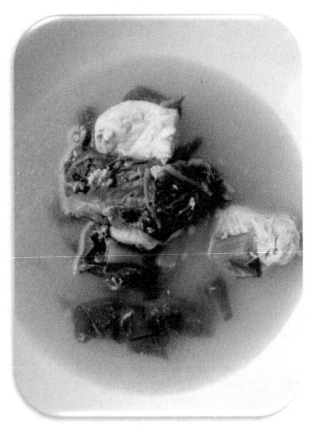

Instructions:

1. In a skillet sauté garlic in olive oil for about 40 seconds. Add the onion and cook for 5 minutes. Season with chili flakes.
2. Add the kale, chicken breast and sauté for 5 minutes.
3. Pour in the chicken stock and bring to a boil. Season with salt, pepper and thyme and cook for 30 minutes.

Spinach Soup (Phase I)

Prep time: 10 minutes

Cooking time: 40 minutes

Servings: 4

Nutrition facts per serving:

Calories 48

Total carbs 3.2 g

Protein 0.7 g

Total sugars 2.2 g

Ingredients:

- 1 cup spinach, chopped
- ¼ cup onion, chopped
- ¼ cup tomatoes, chopped
- 3 garlic cloves, minced
- 1 tbsp butter
- 2 tsp cumin seeds
- 1 tbsp lemon juice
- 3 cups water
- Salt and pepper to taste

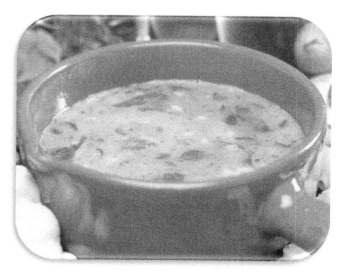

Instructions:

1. In a deep skillet sauté garlic in butter for about 40 seconds. Add the onion, tomatoes, spinach and cumin seeds and cook for 3 minutes. Season with salt and pepper.
2. Pour in the water and bring to a boil. Cook for 15 minutes.

Note: can be enjoyed with cooked rice on Phase II.

Home-style Dal (Phase I)

Prep time: 10 minutes

Cooking time: 40 minutes

Servings: 4

Nutrition facts per serving:

Calories 110

Total carbs 12.3 g

Protein 2.8 g

Total sugars 1.3 g

Ingredients:

- ½ cup garbanzo beans, rinsed
- 1 onion, chopped
- 8-10 fenugreek seeds
- ½ tsp turmeric powder
- Salt and ground coriander to taste
- 1½ tsp cow-milk ghee
- 1 tsp cumin seeds
- 5-6 curry leaves
- 2 green chilies, seeded, chopped
- 1½ cups water

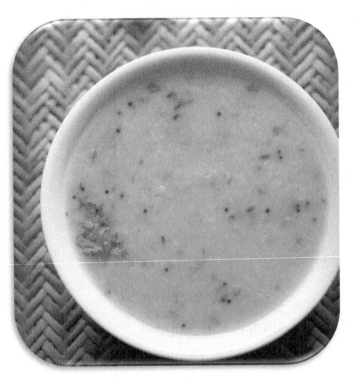

Instructions:

1. Add the rinsed beans to the pressure cooker, pour water. Add turmeric, fenugreek and onion and pressure cook on high for 10 min.
2. In a deep pan heat the ghee, add cumin seeds, curry leaves and chilies.
3. Add the cooked beans and season with salt and coriander. Simmer for 5 minutes. Add water in case you find the dal too thick.

Gazpacho (Phase I/II)

Prep time: 10 minutes

Cooking time: 15 minutes

Servings: 6

Nutrition facts per serving:

Calories 135

Total carbs 12.6 g

Protein 2.9 g

Total sugars 5.5 g

Ingredients:

- 3 red tomatoes, diced
- 3 yellow tomatoes, diced
- 1 cucumber, peeled, diced
- 1 onion, diced
- 2 celery stalks, diced
- 1 red sweet pepper, diced
- 1 tsp minced garlic
- ¼ cup red wine vinegar
- 3 tbsp basil, chopped
- 3 tbsp parsley, chopped
- ¼ cup olive oil
- 2 tbsp lemon juice
- 1 tsp Worcestershire sauce
- 2 cups tomato juice
- Salt and pepper to taste

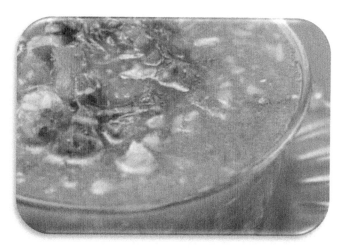

Instructions:

1. In a food processor pulse the tomatoes, garlic and salt until desired consistency.
2. Put red wine vinegar and tomato mixture into a large pot.
3. In a food processor pulse cucumbers and onion. Add to the pot.
4. Repeat with the celery and red pepper. Add to the pot.
5. Add in basil, parsley, olive oil, lemon juice, Worcestershire sauce and tomato juice.
6. Season with pepper and check for consistency. If gazpacho is too thick for you, add more tomato juice.
7. Serve cool.

Split Pea Soup with Italian Sausage
(Phase I/II)

Prep time: 10 minutes

Cooking time: 50 minutes

Servings: 6

Nutrition facts per serving:

Calories 477

Total carbs 49.5 g

Protein 35.5 g

Total sugars 10.6 g

Ingredients:

- 2 cups yellow split peas
- 5 links turkey Italian sausage, cubed
- 1 onion, diced
- 1 cup celery, diced
- 1 green bell pepper, diced
- 1 tbsp minced garlic
- 2 tbsp olive oil
- 1 tsp Italian herb blend
- ½ tsp fennel seeds
- 6 cups chicken stock
- Salt and pepper to taste

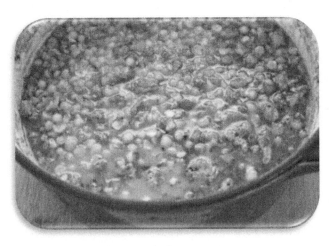

Instructions:

1. In a large pot heat 1 tbsp olive oil and sauté onion, celery and green pepper for 3-4 min.
2. Add garlic, Italian herb blend and fennel seeds to the pot.
3. In a saucepan heat 1 tbsp olive oil and sauté the sausages, breaking them apart, until golden.
4. Add sausages to the pot of vegetables along with the split peas and chicken stock. Season with salt and pepper.
5. Bring to a boil and let simmer until the peas are soft.

Stuffed Peppers Soup (Phase I)

Prep time: 10 minutes

Cooking time: 50 minutes

Servings: 6

Nutrition facts per serving:

Calories 438

Total carbs 28.1 g

Protein 41.7 g

Total sugars 6.3 g

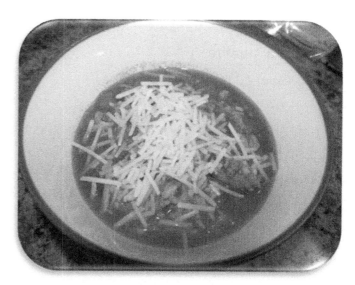

Ingredients:

- 2 green bell peppers, seeded, chopped into ½ inch cubes
- 5 links turkey Italian sausage
- 1 lb ground beef, lean
- 1 onion, chopped
- 2 cans (15 oz) crushed tomatoes
- 4 tsp olive oil
- 1 tbsp Italian herb blend
- 1 tbsp Worcestershire sauce
- ½ cup ketchup
- Salt and pepper to taste
- 7 cups beef stock
- Parmesan cheese for serving

Instructions:

1. In a frying pan heat 2 tsp olive oil and sauté onion until golden. Season with Italian herb blend.
2. Transfer the onions into a large pot.
3. In the same frying pan sauté bell peppers for 3-4 min and add to the pot.
4. Add 2 more tsp olive oil to the frying pan and add the sausages and ground beef. Cook until browned breaking apart as it cooks.
5. Add beef and sausages to the pot.
6. Add the tomatoes, beef broth, Worcestershire sauce, and ketchup and bring to a boil.
7. Let simmer for 40 minutes.
8. Serve hot with Parmesan if desired.

Egg Soup (Phase I)

Prep time: 10 minutes

Cooking time: 50 minutes

Servings: 6

Nutrition facts per serving:

Calories 438

Total carbs 28.1 g

Protein 41.7 g

Total sugars 6.3 g

Ingredients:

- 1 egg
- 1 egg white
- 4 tbsp green onion, chopped
- 2 cups chicken broth
- 2 tsp soy sauce
- Pepper to taste

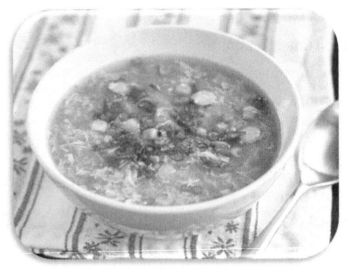

Instructions:

1. In a bowl beat a whole egg with the egg white.
2. Pour the chicken broth into a pot and bring to a boil.
3. Add green onions and remove from the heat.
4. Stir in the beaten egg gradually. Then add soy sauce and season with pepper.
5. Serve hot.

Chinese Hot and Sour Soup (Phase I)

Prep time: 10 minutes

Cooking time: 50 minutes

Servings: 5

Nutrition facts per serving:

Calories 90

Total carbs 3.4 g

Protein 13.4 g

Total sugars 1.6 g

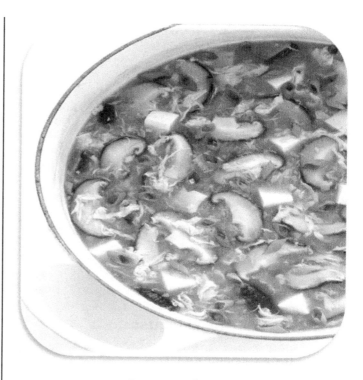

Ingredients:

- 4 oz chicken breast, cooked, cut into strips
- ½ cup mushrooms, sliced
- 1 egg, beaten
- 1 tsp minced ginger
- 1/3 cup bamboo shoots, canned, cut into strips
- ¼ cup scallions, chopped
- 1/3 cup fresh snow pea pods
- ¼ cup rice vinegar
- ¼ cup soy sauce, low carb
- ½ tsp hot sauce
- 5 cups chicken broth
- Salt and pepper to taste

Instructions:

1. In a large pot combine chicken broth, mushrooms and ginger and bring to a boil.
2. Add chicken strips and let simmer for 10 minutes.
3. Add bamboo shoots and simmer for 5 minutes.
4. Add vinegar, soy sauce and hot sauce and bring to a boil again.
5. Add scallions and snow peas and cook for 1 minute. Take off the heat.
6. Slowly stir in the egg.
7. Season with pepper and top with more scallions, if desired.

Creamy Celery Cheddar Soup (Phase I)

Prep time: 10 minutes

Cooking time: 50 minutes

Servings: 4

Nutrition facts per serving:

Calories 335

Total carbs 14.3 g

Protein 18 g

Total sugars 5.7 g

Ingredients:

- 3 tomatoes, chopped
- 1 celery stalk, chopped
- 2 green onions, chopped
- 1 tsp basil
- ¼ tsp onion powder
- 1 cup half & half
- 3 cups chicken stock
- 1½ cups Cheddar, shredded
- Salt and pepper to taste

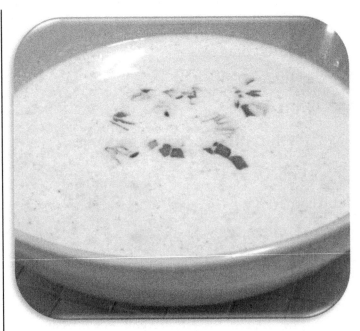

Instructions:

1. In a food processor combine and purée 1 cup chicken stock, tomatoes, celery and green onions.
2. Pour 2 cups chicken stock into a soup pot and bring to a boil.
3. Add the processed vegetables and bring to a boil again.
4. Stir in half & half and season with basil, onion powder, salt and pepper.
5. Let simmer for 5 minutes, then add cheese and stir until melted.

Fish & Seafood

Pecan Crusted Cod (Phase I)

Prep time: 10 minutes

Cooking time: 20 minutes

Servings: 4

Nutrition facts per serving:

Calories 228

Total carbs 2.2 g

Protein 22.3 g

Total sugars 0.6 g

Ingredients:

- 4 cod fillets
- ¼ cup pecans, roasted
- 1 garlic clove
- 1 egg white, beaten
- 1 tsp red chili powder
- 1 tsp dried rosemary
- 2 tbsp olive oil
- Salt to taste

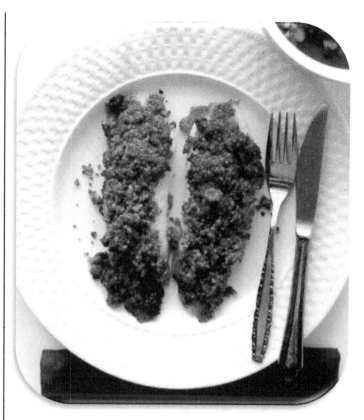

Instructions:

1. In a food processor finely chop the pecans, rosemary, garlic and chili powder.
2. Preheat the oven to 400°F.
3. Place the fish fillets on a baking sheet and season with salt. Brush with egg white and sprinkle with nut mixture.
4. Bake about 20 minutes.

Balsamic Salmon (Phase I/II)

Prep time: 10 minutes

Cooking time: 30 minutes

Servings: 2

Nutrition facts per serving:

Calories 306

Total carbs 8.1 g

Protein 43.5 g

Total sugars 0.6 g

Ingredients:

- 2 salmon fillets
- ½ cup balsamic vinegar
- ½ tsp lemon juice
- 1 tsp olive oil
- Salt and pepper to taste

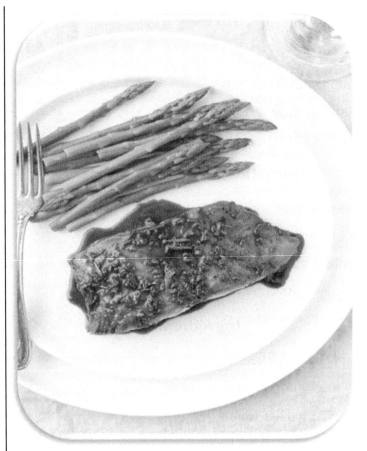

Instructions:

1. Preheat the oven to 450°F.
2. Season the fish fillets with salt and pepper, and place in a baking dish. Cover with foil. Bake for 15 minutes.
3. Prepare the balsamic glaze by stirring the vinegar over medium heat until reduced by about two-thirds. Add the lemon juice and olive oil.
4. Coat the salmon with glaze and serve.
5. Serve with asparagus for Phase I or with cooked rice for Phase II.

Cedar Plank Salmon (Phase I)

Prep time: 5 minutes

Cooking time: 20 minutes

Servings: 2

Nutrition facts per serving:

Calories 438

Total carbs 10.6 g

Protein 42.4 g

Total sugars 9.3 g

Ingredients:

- 2 salmon fillets
- 1 tsp cumin powder
- 1 tsp smoked paprika
- ½ tsp dried thyme
- ½ tsp garlic powder
- 1 tbsp olive oil
- Salt and pepper to taste

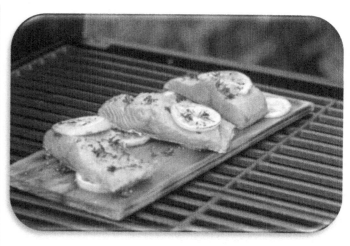

Instructions:

1. Prepare the grill by soaking cedar planks in water for at least 1 hour and preheating the grill.
2. In a bowl mix all dry ingredients and 1 tbsp olive oil. Combine to make a paste and rub it all over the salmon.
3. Place the fish on cedar planks and arrange on a grill over medium heat.
4. Cover and smoke for 20 minutes.

Tilapia Ceviche (Phase I)

Prep time: 3 hours

Cooking time: 10 minutes

Servings: 4

Nutrition facts per serving:

Calories 87

Total carbs 9.9 g

Protein 13 g

Total sugars 3.4 g

Ingredients:

- 2 tilapia fillets, diced
- 2 Roma tomatoes, diced
- 3 limes, juiced
- ½ onion, diced
- ½ tsp red chili garlic paste
- 2½ tbsp cilantro, chopped
- Salt and pepper to taste

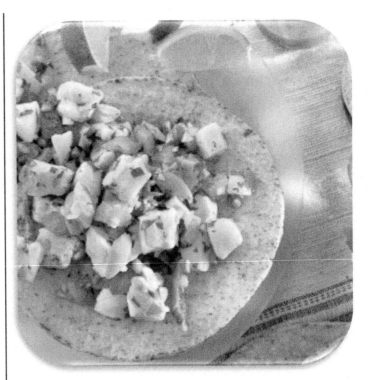

Instructions:

1. Marinate the diced fish fillets in lime juice for 3 hours in the refrigerator.
2. Drain the liquid from the fish and set it aside. Mix the chili paste, tomatoes, onion and some of the lime juice, and then mix it with the fish. Season with salt and pepper.

Note: can be served with tortilla chips for Phase II.

Bok Choy Shrimp (Phase I)

Prep time: 5 minutes

Cooking time: 20 minutes

Servings: 4

Nutrition facts per serving:

Calories 95

Total carbs 3.9 g

Protein 10.1 g

Total sugars 1.6 g

Ingredients:

- 20 shrimp, cleaned, deveined
- 3 bok choy bunches, chopped, use both stalks and leaves
- 1 onion, sliced
- 1 tbsp olive oil
- 1 tbsp soy sauce
- 2 garlic cloves, minced
- 2 tsp red chili flakes
- Salt and pepper to taste

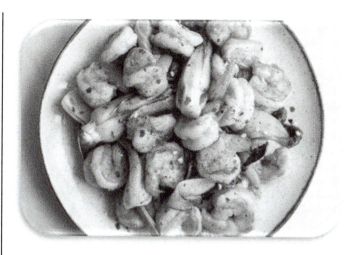

Instructions:

1. In a skillet sauté garlic in olive oil for 30 seconds. Add onions and chili flakes and cook for 2-3 minutes more.
2. Add the shrimp and cook for 5 minutes.
3. After 5 minutes remove the shrimp and add the bok choy and soy sauce and cook for 5 minutes or until tender.
4. Season with salt and pepper and add shrimp back to the pan.
5. Stir and serve.

Chipotle Shrimp with Zucchini Noodles (Phase I)

Prep time: 15 minutes

Cooking time: 8 minutes

Servings: 4

Nutrition facts per serving:

Calories 316

Total carbs 10.4 g

Protein 43.6 g

Total sugars 2.4 g

Ingredients:

- 20 shrimp, cleaned, deveined
- 2 chipotle peppers
- 1 tbsp Adobo sauce
- 1 tbsp agave syrup
- 2 tbsp olive oil + 1 tsp for sautéing
- 2 garlic cloves
- ½ tsp cumin powder
- 1 tsp oregano
- 3 zucchini, spiralized
- Salt and pepper to taste

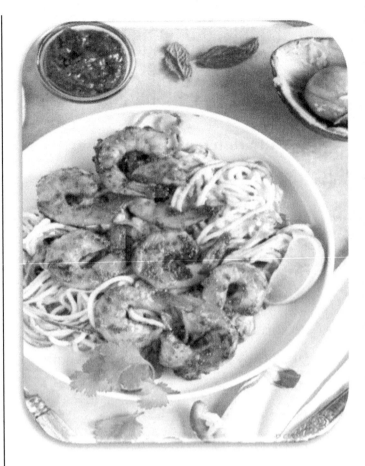

Instructions:

1. In a food processor blend chipotles, adobo, 1 tbsp olive oil, 1 tbsp agave syrup, 2 garlic cloves, cumin powder and oregano.
2. Coat shrimp in the chipotle sauce.
3. In a skillet sauté the zucchini in olive oil, season with salt and pepper.
4. Remove the cooked zucchini from the pan and add the marinated shrimp to the same pan. Cook for 2-3 minutes on each side.

Red Fish Stew (Phase I/II)

Prep time: 15 minutes

Cooking time: 30 minutes

Servings: 6

Nutrition facts per serving:

Calories 335

Total carbs 7.1 g

Protein 55.1 g

Total sugars 4.4 g

Ingredients:

- 8 (10 oz) cod, tilapia or halibut fillets, cut into 1 inch cubes
- ½ cup red onion, chopped
- 12 oz red bell peppers, chopped
- 1 can (14.5 oz) tomatoes, diced, with juice
- 1 tsp minced garlic
- 1 tbsp olive oil
- ¼ tsp red pepper flakes
- ¼ cup fresh cilantro, chopped
- ½ tsp lemon zest, grated
- 2 tsp lemon juice
- Salt and pepper to taste

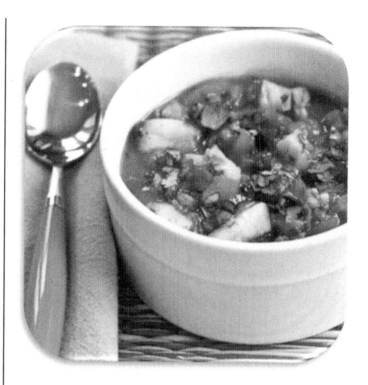

Instructions:

1. In a skillet sauté onion in olive oil for 3-4 minutes. Add bell peppers, tomatoes with juice, garlic and red pepper flakes. Add some water if more liquid is required.
2. Let simmer for 10 minutes.
3. Add lemon juice and zest and ¼ cup cilantro.
4. Add fish and stir to combine.
5. Season with salt and pepper and let simmer for 10 minutes.
6. Serve with fresh cilantro.

Note: can be enjoyed with cooked rice for Phase II.

Almond and Parmesan Baked Fish (Phase I/II)

Prep time: 15 minutes

Cooking time: 30 minutes

Servings: 4

Nutrition facts per serving:

Calories 189

Total carbs 1 g

Protein 18.8 g

Total sugars 0.2 g

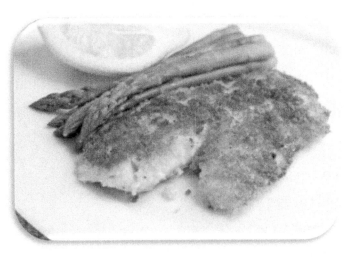

Ingredients:

- 4 white fish fillets, ½ inch thick
- 1/3 cup almond meal
- ¼ cup butter, melted
- 2 tbsp Parmesan, grated
- ½ tsp garlic powder
- Salt and pepper to taste
- ½ tsp fish rub

Instructions:

1. Preheat oven to 425°F.
2. In a bowl mix the almond meal, Parmesan, garlic powder, salt, pepper and fish rub.
3. Coat the fillets with butter all over; then dip into the almond meal mixture.
4. Bake for 20-30 minutes.

Fish & Cabbage Bowls (Phase I/II)

Prep time: 15 minutes

Cooking time: 30 minutes

Servings: 4

Nutrition facts per serving:

Calories 178

Total carbs 13 g

Protein 15.5 g

Total sugars 7.6 g

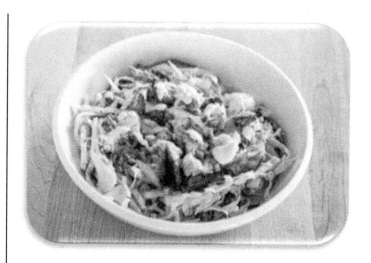

Ingredients:

- 3 white fish fillets
- 1 head green cabbage, sliced thin
- ½ head red cabbage, sliced thin
- ½ cup green onions, sliced
- 4 tsp olive oil
- 2 tsp fish rub
- 1 tsp ground cumin
- ½ tsp chili powder
- 1/2 cup mix of mayonnaise and plain Greek yogurt
- 2 tbsp lime juice
- 2 tsp green Tabasco Sauce
- Salt and pepper to taste

Instructions:

1. Mix together fish rub, ground cumin, and chili powder.
2. Rub the fish fillets with olive oil and dip into fish rub mixture.
3. Prepare the dressing by mixing mayo, Greek yogurt, lime juice and green Tabasco Sauce. Season with salt and pepper.
4. Preheat a frying pan with 2 tsp olive oil and cook fish on both sides for 8-10 minutes total.
5. Mix half the green onions with the green and red cabbage and stir in some dressing to moisten the cabbage.
6. When the fish is done, shred it apart with a fork.
7. Arrange the cabbage mixture in a bowl and top with fish. Drizzle over some dressing.
8. Serve with the remaining green onions.

Shrimp Cocktail

Prep time: 5 minutes

Cooking time: 15 minutes

Servings: 6

Nutrition facts per serving:

Calories 85

Total carbs 4.3 g

Protein 13.7 g

Total sugars 2.6 g

Ingredients:

- 30 shrimp, boiled and peeled
- 1/2 cup low-sugar ketchup
- 2 tbsp tomato paste
- 3 tsp lemon juice
- 4 tsp cream-style horseradish

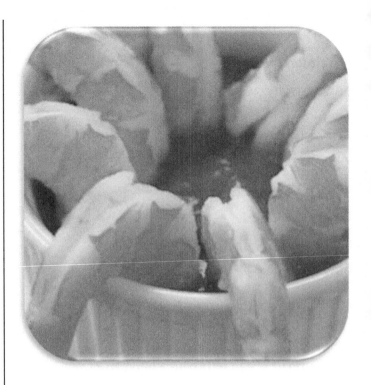

Instructions:

1. Stir together tomato paste and ketchup, add lemon juice and horseradish.
2. Serve shrimp with the cocktail sauce.

Salmon Cucumber Bites (Phase II)

Prep time: 5 minutes

Cooking time: none

Servings: 2

Nutrition facts per serving:

Calories 110

Total carbs 4 g

Protein 10 g

Total sugars 2.6 g

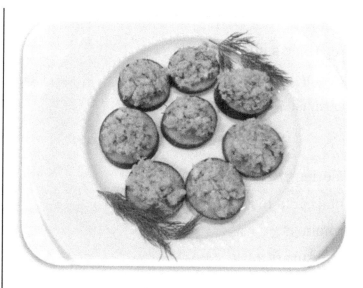

Ingredients:

- 3 oz pink salmon, canned
- 16 slices cucumber
- 1 tbsp celery, minced
- 1 tbsp onion, minced
- 1 tbsp mayonnaise
- ½ tsp yellow mustard
- 1 tsp fresh dill

Instructions:

1. Combine all ingredients except the cucumbers and stir.
2. Spoon salmon mixture on each cucumber slice and serve.

Spicy Mussels

Prep time: 5 minutes

Cooking time: 15 minutes

Servings: 4

Nutrition facts per serving:

Calories 370

Total carbs 16 g

Protein 37 g

Total sugars 2.6 g

Ingredients:

- 4 lb mussels, beards removed
- 1 cup canned tomatoes, crushed
- 3 garlic cloves, minced
- 1 onion, chopped
- 2 tbsp olive oil
- 1 tsp basil, dried
- ¼ tsp red pepper flakes
- ½ cup water

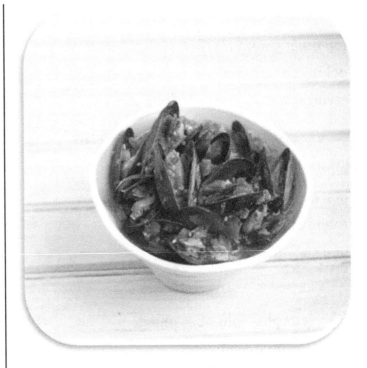

Instructions:

1. In a large skillet sauté onion, garlic and basil in olive oil for 3-4 min. Add pepper flakes.
2. Add water and bring to a boil, let simmer for 3 minutes.
3. Add tomatoes and mussels and cover. Cook for 8 minutes or until the mussels open.

Poultry

Turkey Roll-ups (Phase I)

Prep time: 5 minutes

Cooking time: 5 minutes

Servings: 4

Nutrition facts per serving:

Calories 126

Total carbs 16.8 g

Protein 9.1 g

Total sugars 8.1 g

Ingredients:

- 4 slices cooked turkey breast
- 4 lettuce leaves
- 4 scallions, diced
- 1 bell pepper, diced
- 4 small cucumbers, diced
- ¾ cup mayonnaise, low fat
- ¾ cup cilantro leaves, chopped
- 1 tbsp lime juice
- 1 tsp soy sauce
- 1 garlic clove, minced

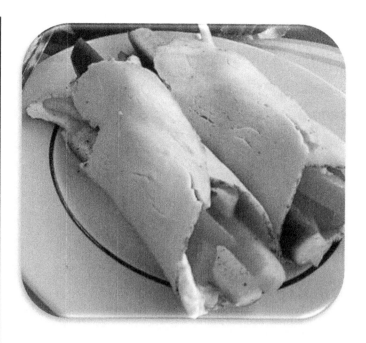

Instructions:

1. In a bowl mix mayo, cilantro, lime juice, soy sauce and garlic.
2. On each turkey slice, spread cilantro mayonnaise mixture, and then layer with lettuce, scallions, cucumber and peppers. Sprinkle with some more cilantro mayo mix and roll.

Pesto Chicken Breasts (Phase I/II)

Prep time: 5 minutes

Cooking time: 50 minutes

Servings: 4

Nutrition facts per serving:

Calories 287

Total carbs 4.3 g

Protein 30.3 g

Total sugars 1.8 g

Ingredients:

- 4 chicken breasts, skinless
- 6 tbsp pesto
- 1 tomato, sliced
- 7 oz mozzarella cheese, grated
- 1 tbsp fresh parsley, chopped
- 1 tbsp fresh basil, chopped
- Salt and pepper to taste

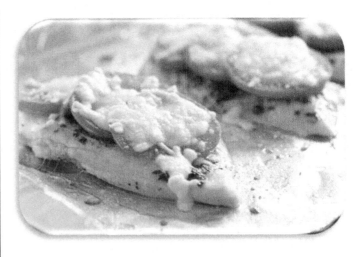

Instructions:

1. Preheat the oven to 355°F.
2. Season the chicken breasts with pesto and salt and pepper.
3. Place into a baking dish and bake for 30 minutes.
4. Take the chicken out and sprinkle with mozzarella, tomatoes, basil and parsley, then mozzarella again.
5. Place the chicken back in oven for 20 more minutes.

Baked Chicken Cordon Bleu (Phase I)

Prep time: 15 minutes

Cooking time: 35 minutes

Servings: 4

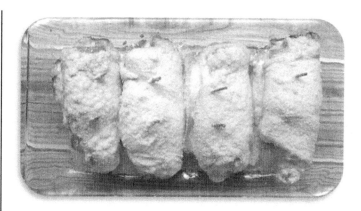

Nutrition facts per serving:

Calories 294

Total carbs 1.7 g

Protein 42.1 g

Total sugars 1.1 g

Ingredients:

- 4 chicken breasts, skinless, halved into 1/3 inch thick pieces
- 8 slices boiled ham
- 2 oz mozzarella, shredded
- 1 egg
- 1 tbsp margarine, melted
- 1/3 cup Parmesan, grated
- Salt and pepper to taste

Instructions:

1. Preheat the oven to 355°F.
2. In a baking dish place one slice ham on a chicken breast half and top with some mozzarella.
3. Roll up and pin with a toothpick.
4. Repeat the layering with the remaining slices.
5. Beat an egg and mix with melted margarine. Season with salt and pepper. Pour over chicken rolls.
6. Sprinkle with grated Parmesan.
7. Bake for 35 minutes.
8. Serve sliced.

Chicken Breasts with Goat Cheese Stuffing (Phase I)

Prep time: 15 minutes

Cooking time: 20 minutes

Servings: 2

Nutrition facts per serving:

Calories 354

Total carbs 4.4 g

Protein 47.9 g

Total sugars 1.1 g

Ingredients:

- 2 chicken breasts, skinless, boneless
- 2 oz goat cheese, low fat
- 1 garlic clove, minced
- ½ bunch spinach
- 2 tsp olive oil
- Salt and pepper to taste

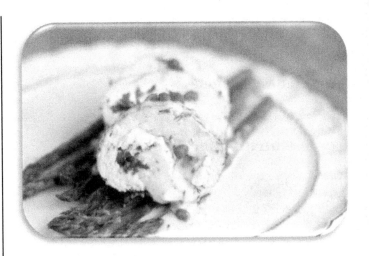

Instructions:

1. In a skillet sauté garlic in 1 tsp olive oil for 3 min.
2. Add spinach and cook for 3-4 minutes. Season with salt and pepper.
3. Cut out a pocket in each chicken breast and fill with spinach and cheese. Season breasts with salt and pepper.
4. Heat 1 tsp olive oil in the skillet and brown the chicken for 5 minutes.
5. Preheat the oven to 400°F. Transfer the chicken to a baking dish.
6. Bake for 10 minutes.

Greek style Chicken (Phase I/II)

Prep time: 2 hours

Cooking time: 20 minutes

Servings: 4

Nutrition facts per serving:

Calories 203

Total carbs 2.2 g

Protein 36.3 g

Total sugars 0.4 g

Ingredients:

- 1.5 lb chicken breasts, skinless
- 1 tbsp rosemary
- 1 tbsp oregano
- ½ tsp smoked paprika
- 4 tbsp lemon juice
- Salt and pepper to taste

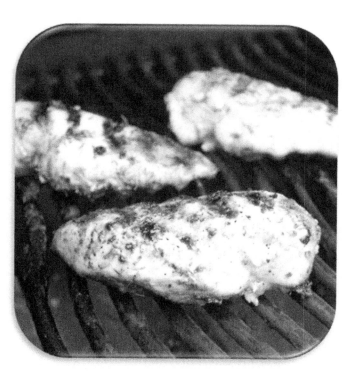

Instructions:

1. Season the chicken with spices and lemon juice and marinate for 2 hours.
2. Arrange the chicken on a grill and cook on each side until browned.

Ground Chicken and Chickpea Stew (Phase I/II)

Prep time: 5 minutes

Cooking time: 30 minutes

Servings: 6

Nutrition facts per serving:

Calories 379

Total carbs 57.7 g

Protein 30.8 g

Total sugars 44.3 g

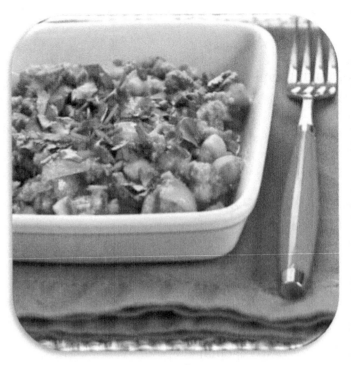

Ingredients:

- 1.5 lb ground chicken or turkey
- 1 onion, chopped
- 1 can (14.5 oz) tomatoes with juice, diced
- 1 can (16 oz) chickpeas
- 12 oz Greek yogurt, fat free
- 1 tbsp + 1 tsp olive oil
- 2 tbsp sweet curry powder
- Salt and pepper to taste

Instructions:

1. In a skillet heat 1 tbsp olive oil and add ground chicken or turkey breaking it apart as it cooks. Cook for about 8 minutes.
2. Add 1 tsp olive oil and chopped onion. Season with curry powder.
3. Add tomatoes with juice and chickpeas. Let simmer until the liquid evaporates.
4. Stir in yogurt and simmer for 3 more minutes.
5. Season with salt and pepper.

Saffron Chicken (Phase I/II)

Prep time: 5 minutes

Cooking time: 1 hour 10 minutes

Servings: 2

Nutrition facts per serving:

Calories 281

Total carbs 9.8 g

Protein 30.7 g

Total sugars 4.1 g

Ingredients:

- 2 chicken breasts, skinless, cut into large cubes
- 1 onion, cut into slices lengthwise
- 1 tbsp olive oil
- 1.5 tbsp lemon juice
- 1 tsp butter
- ¾ cup chicken stock
- Pinch saffron
- Salt and pepper to taste
- ¼ cup parsley, chopped

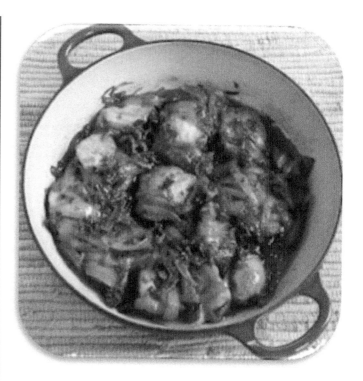

Instructions:

1. In a skillet brown the chicken in olive oil and butter.
2. Remove the chicken and add the onions to the pan; brown until golden over low heat.
3. Return chicken to the pan and cover with onions.
4. Add the stock and saffron, bring to a boil and let simmer for 45 minutes covered.
5. Add lemon juice, parsley and water if needed. Let simmer for 10 minutes.

Ground Turkey Lettuce Wraps
(Phase I/II)

Prep time: 5 minutes

Cooking time: 1 hour 10 minutes

Servings: 6

Nutrition facts per serving:

Calories 174

Total carbs 5.7 g

Protein 28.4 g

Total sugars 2.3 g

Ingredients:

- 1.5 lb ground turkey
- 1 large head lettuce
- 3 tbsp onions, chopped
- 2 tbsp ginger root, grated
- 2 tbsp garlic, minced
- 1 tbsp olive oil
- 4 tbsp soy sauce
- 1 tbsp chili garlic sauce
- 1 cup cilantro, chopped

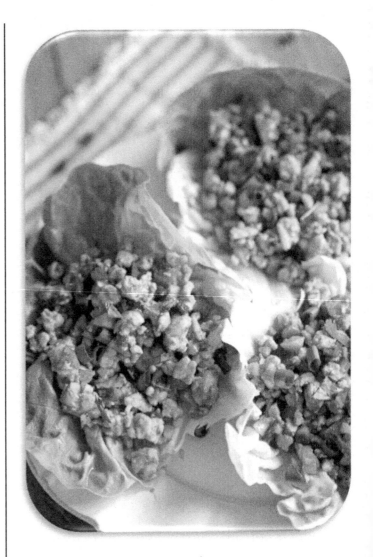

Instructions:

1. In a skillet sauté onions in olive oil for 2-3 minutes, add garlic and ginger root and sauté for 1 more minute.
2. Add ground turkey, breaking it apart as it cooks.
3. Add soy sauce and chili garlic sauce and cook until the turkey is brown.
4. Add chopped cilantro.
5. Take a lettuce leaf and fill it with turkey mixture and fold.

Asian Marinade Kebabs (Phase I/II)

Prep time: overnight

Cooking time: 20 minutes

Servings: 4

Nutrition facts per serving:

Calories 321

Total carbs 4.7 g

Protein 29.8 g

Total sugars 1.7 g

Ingredients:

- 4 chicken breasts, skinless, cut crosswise and cubed
- ¼ cup olive oil
- ¼ cup soy sauce
- 1 tbsp Asian sesame oil
- 1 tbsp garlic, minced
- 2 tsp ginger, grated
- 3 tbsp lime juice
- 1 tsp curry powder
- Salt and pepper to taste

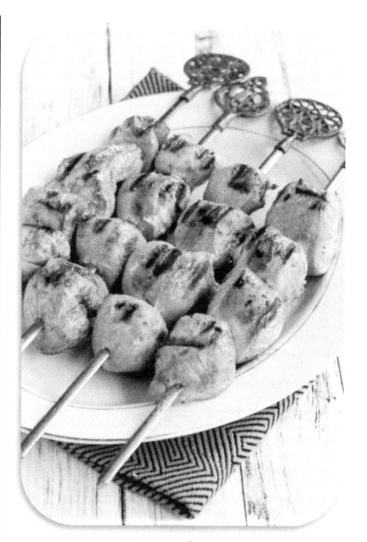

Instructions:

1. Make the marinade by mixing together olive oil, soy sauce, sesame oil, minced garlic, grated ginger, fresh lime juice, and curry powder.
2. Add chicken to a zip-lock bag and pour over the marinade. Marinate for 6-10 hours in the fridge.
3. Thread the chicken onto skewers and cook on a grill for 10 minutes.
4. Turn the skewers over and grill 5 minutes more.
5. Serve hot.

Tarragon Mustard Chicken (Phase I/II)

Prep time: overnight

Cooking time: 15 minutes

Servings: 4

Nutrition facts per serving:

Calories 317

Total carbs 1.4 g

Protein 29 g

Total sugars 0.1 g

Ingredients:

- 4 chicken breasts, skinless, cut in half
- 1/3 cup olive oil
- 2 tbsp tarragon, chopped
- 2 tbsp Dijon mustard
- 1 tbsp fresh lemon juice
- 1 tsp minced garlic or garlic purée
- 1 tsp Spike Seasoning

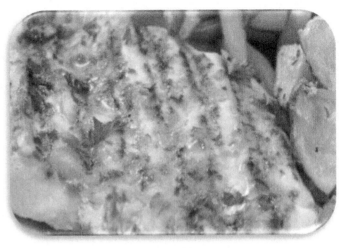

Instructions:

1. In a food processor make the marinade by blending together tarragon, olive oil, mustard, lemon juice, garlic and Spike Seasoning.
2. Add chicken to a zip-lock bag and pour over the marinade. Marinate for 6-10 hours in the fridge.
3. Lay chicken breasts onto a preheated grill and cook, rotating, until chicken is browned and firm.
4. Serve hot.

Charmoula Sauce Chicken (Phase I/II)

Prep time: overnight

Cooking time: 15 minutes

Servings: 4

Nutrition facts per serving:

Calories 295

Total carbs 2.1 g

Protein 29.4 g

Total sugars 0.7 g

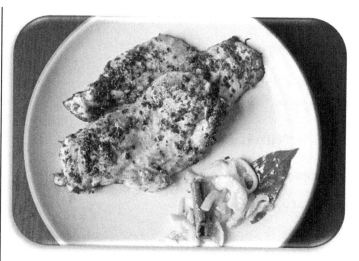

Ingredients:

- 4 chicken breasts, skinless, cut in half crosswise
- 2 garlic cloves, chopped
- 1/2 cup cilantro, chopped
- 1/4 cup parsley, chopped
- 1 tbsp + 2 tsp lemon juice
- 1/2 tsp sweet paprika
- 1/2 tsp ground cumin
- 4 tbsp olive oil
- Salt and pepper to taste

Instructions:

1. Make the marinade by blending together chopped garlic, chopped cilantro, chopped parsley, lemon juice, sweet paprika, and ground cumin.
2. Add chicken to a zip-lock bag and pour over the marinade. Marinate for 6-10 hours in the fridge.
3. You can fry the chicken in a preheated pan or grill it on a preheated grill on all sides until golden.

Spinach Stuffed Chicken

Prep time: 5 minutes

Cooking time: 1 hour

Servings: 4

Nutrition facts per serving:

Calories 308

Total carbs 9 g

Protein 32 g

Total sugars 0.7 g

Ingredients:

- 4 chicken breasts, skinless
- 12 oz frozen spinach soufflé, cut into 4 equal parts
- 2 garlic cloves, sliced
- 2 tbsp olive oil
- 1 tsp Dijon mustard
- 2 tbsp lemon juice
- 1 cup chicken stock
- Salt and pepper to taste

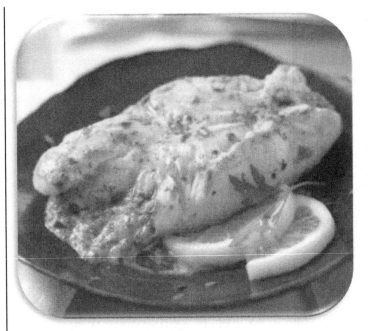

Instructions:

1. Top half of each chicken breast with spinach soufflé piece. Fold half of the chicken over the filling and pin with wooden picks.
2. In a skillet sauté garlic in olive oil until golden.
3. Remove the garlic and brown the chicken breasts for 7 minutes on each side.
4. Preheat the oven to 350°F.
5. Place the chicken onto a baking dish and bake for 40 minutes.
6. In a sauce pan heat the stock, lemon juice, mustard, salt and pepper. Add back the garlic. Bring to a boil and let simmer for 20 minutes.
7. Serve the chicken with the sauce, garnished with parsley.

Recipe Index

CONCLUSION

Thank you for reading this book and having the patience to try these recipes.

I do hope that you gain as much enjoyment reading and experimenting with the meals as I have had writing this books.

If you would like to leave a comment, you can do it at the Order section->Digital orders, in your amazon account.

Stay safe and healthy!

Conversion Tables

VALUME EQUIVALENTS (LIQUID)

US STANDARD	US STANDARD (OUNCES)	METRIC (% PROXIMATE)
2 tablespoons	1 fl. oz.	30 mL
¼ cup	2 fl. oz.	60 mL
½ cup	4 fl. oz.	120 mL
1 cup	8 fl. oz.	240mL
1 ½ cup	12 fl. oz.	355 mL
2 cups or 1 pint	16 fl. oz.	475 mL
4 cups or 1 quart	32 fl. oz.	1 L
1 gallon	128 fl. oz.	4 L

OVEN TEMPERATURES

FAHRENHEIT(F)	CELSIUS(C) APPROXIMATE
250 °F	120 °C
300 °F	150 °C
325 °F	165 °C
350 °F	180 °C
375 °F	190°C
400 °F	200 °C
425 °F	220 °C
450 °F	230 °C

VALUME EQUIVALENTS (LIQUID)

US STANDARD	METRIC (APPROXIMATE)
$\frac{1}{8}$ teaspoon	0.5 mL
¼ teaspoon	1 mL
½ teaspoon	2 mL
$\frac{2}{3}$ teaspoon	4 mL
1 teaspoon	5 mL
1 tablespoon	15 mL
¼ cup	59 mL
$\frac{1}{3}$ cup	79 mL
½ cup	118 mL
$\frac{2}{3}$ cup	156 mL
¾ cup	177 mL
1 cup	235 mL
2 cups or 1 pint	475 mL
3 cups	700 mL
4 cups or 1 quart	1 L
½ gallon	2 L
1 gallon	4 L

WEIGHT EQUIVALENTS

US STANDARD	METRIC (APPROXIMATE)
½ ounce	15 g
1 ounces	30 g
2 ounces	60 g
4 ounces	115 g
8 ounces	225 g
12 ounces	340 g
16 ounce or 1 pound	455 g

Other Books by Emma Green

Intermittent Fasting https://goo.gl/i4WMva

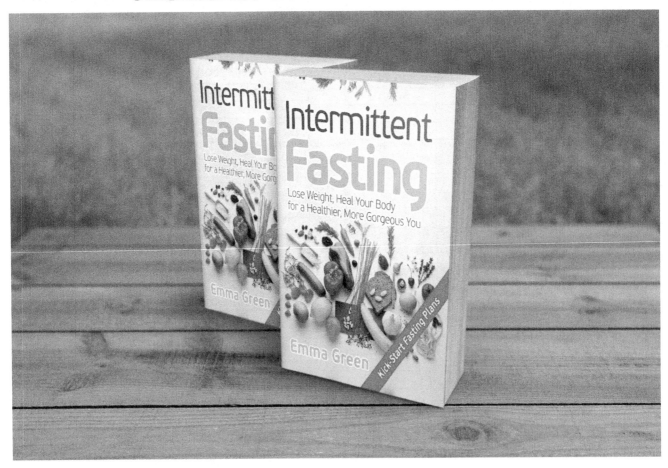

Made in the USA
Middletown, DE
11 October 2018